# THE DIAGNOSTIC INTERVIEW

# THE DIAGNOSTIC INTERVIEW

*Second Edition*

## Ian Stevenson, M.D.

ALUMNI PROFESSOR OF PSYCHIATRY,
DEPARTMENT OF PSYCHIATRY,
UNIVERSITY OF VIRGINIA SCHOOL OF MEDICINE,
CHARLOTTESVILLE

MEDICAL DEPARTMENT
HARPER & ROW, PUBLISHERS
NEW YORK, EVANSTON, SAN FRANCISCO, AND LONDON

THE DIAGNOSTIC INTERVIEW

Copyright © 1960, 1971 by Harper & Row, Publishers, Inc.,
All rights reserved. No part of this book may be used
or reproduced in any manner whatsoever without written
permission except in the case of brief quotations
embodied in critical articles and reviews. Printed in
the United States of America. For information address
Medical Department, Harper & Row, Publishers, Inc.,
49 East 33rd Street, New York, N.Y. 10016

First Edition
Standard Book Number 06-142501-X
Library of Congress Catalog Card Number: 72-133141

First Edition published under the title MEDICAL HISTORY-TAKING

*Should I let students take the journals home?* You can keep better control of the process by not letting students take their journals home. You also avoid the possibility that confidentiality will be breached. Students should not think of journal writing as homework. Allow students time in class to write in their journals. By controlling the amount of time students have to write in their journals, you can better manage your responses.

*What if students want to know how to spell a word?* Since the purpose of dialogue journals is to promote fluency in writing, let children spell the words the way they sound. Students won't take risks in their journal writing if they are afraid of making spelling mistakes. Do not circle spelling errors. In your response you can model the correct spelling of the word.

*What about grading the journals?* Dialogue journals are not intended to be graded. The purpose of the journal is to build fluency in writing and to establish a relationship with another person in print.

of, but voice your own opinion if you don't agree. Focus on your students' interests or things you have noticed them talking about or reading in their free time. A simple question such as, "What do you like about the main character in that book?" might motivate students to respond by writing about a book they recently have read.

*How often should I write in the students' journals?* This will depend on your personal schedule. Collecting the journals once a week is a good target to shoot for, but you could also stagger them and take half the class's journals at the end of one week and the other half the next week. To start out, you might try collecting the journals every other day and see how that goes. The number of students in your class and the amount of time available will determine to some extent how often you can write responses.

*How long should my journal entry be?* Try not to make your entry longer than the student's entry. Especially in the beginning, don't overwhelm the student with too much reading.

*What about the issue of student privacy?* At the outset, students should know that their journal is a private place to write and that nothing they write will be made public without their consent. If student confidentiality is respected, then students will come to trust you.

*When should students be given time to read my responses to their journal entries?* If you collect journals every week, or every other day, give students time in the morning for them to read your comments. You will find that the students will look forward to your comments as much as you look forward to theirs.

*Will dialogue journals work with all students?* Some students may not enjoy journal writing as much as others. They may complain that they have nothing to write about or that they are tired of writing. Don't force them to write, but keep writing to them about your interests or things that might appeal to them.

# Practical Considerations in Using Dialogue Journals

Teachers might have many questions about implementing dialogue journals in the classroom: How do you begin? What do students write about? What about the issue of student privacy? These and other questions are covered in this chapter.

*How do I get started?* A good way to introduce students to the idea of dialogue journals is to photocopy your own personal entry in a journal and distribute it to the entire class. This can serve as a model for the type of entries students can write. They might want to begin by writing a response to your entry in their journals, or they can refer to information in your entry that is pertinent to their own entry.

Spiral notebooks work best for keeping entries in order. Tell students to write on one side of the paper. The response from you or another student can be written on the other side. Make it clear to students that this kind of writing is not intended to be a theme such as they might write in an English class. Rather, tell them that dialogue journals will provide an opportunity for you to "talk" privately with each of them.

*What should I as a teacher write in a journal?* When responding to students' journal entries, write honest responses with genuine personalized questions. Write about a similar experience that you have had, or try to put what students have written in a different perspective. Try to get students to elaborate. Agree with things you approve

> *I want to implement this idea into my classroom. Dialogue journals allow children to express themselves more, when otherwise they may not.*
>
> *Hello. Well this is the last dialogue journal that I will have to write for this class. I think it was a good idea because it was the only "personal" means of communication we had with one another. I plan to use dialogue journals in my own classrooms because I feel it breaks down the barrier often found between students and teachers. I know it helped me get to know you a little better.*
>
> *Thanks for writing to me. I really like this idea. Your writing helps me understand things a little better.*
>
> *I'd like to comment on these journals. At the beginning of the semester, I thought it would be a pain trying to come up with ideas to write about. I realize now what a benefit they are. It has given me a chance to express my personal experiences and attitudes. I have always preferred to write than to speak in class. It has also given me a chance to receive feedback, which I thoroughly enjoy. It is nice getting other people's opinions.*
>
> *I write some poetry in my personal journal. Most of the time that is just a release for me. Writing in my journal is a way to get all my feelings out, sorted, collected and then try and figure what's going on.*

As students write more in their journals, they become more confident in their ability to write, and they are more comfortable writing. By reading their own writing and responding to someone else's writing, students become more fluent in making meaning from the written word.

# Developing Fluency in Writing Through Dialogue Journals

Students' writing in dialogue journals is much like conversation in print. It is a natural form of writing, because students are writing for a purpose and are responding to another person's writing. As students continue to write in their journals, their entries become longer and their sentence structures become more complex. When composing their own thoughts and responding to the comments and questions of others, students learn to manipulate language in new ways. They are developing fluency in writing.

Dialogue journals provide teachers with an ideal means for watching the writing development of individual students. Teachers can identify writing problems in language mechanics and usage, which later can become the basis for direct instruction for individuals or groups.

Teachers have observed that children's invented spelling often becomes standard spelling as the children see their teachers model correct spelling in their journal entries. The journals also serve as a source for developing "demon" spelling lists for individual students.

Students also report the benefits of dialogue journals. Following are excerpts from journals of students in a college education class in which they comment on the benefits of dialogue journals:

*Journal*

*I feel that the idea of dialogue journals is great. As I stated in my paper, we also did them in high school. Depending on the grade level I'm teaching,*

*Desendre 11 1985*
*Mommy*
   *Is that Wrd I Well HaV Mor spaces. IN MY Mawth I do Not Lik lim sumtims OK Now tim for my dey It was a fun Dey I HaD too Dey My GeNGgrBriED Man ran Ha wat Man and ran rim OK Lets Git Bak too MY Dey OK War Was I My GeNGrBrieD Man ran a wa Lat Was Fane I DoNt NO Wat els too sa so I ges I wel go Naw BY BY*

*Love, Ann*

(Translation of Ann's entry: "December 11, 1985. Mommy, Is that weird. I will have more spaces in my mouth. I do not like them sometimes. OK, now time for my day. It was a fun day I had today. My gingerbread man ran. Hey wait, man and ran rhyme. OK let's get back to my day. OK where was I? My gingerbread man ran away. That was funny. I don't know what else to say so I guess I will go now. Bye Bye. Love, Ann.")

In her own way, Ann is learning about language as she carries on a conversation with her mother in her journal. In addition to her printed messages, she includes drawings and other decorative elements, which add to the fun of the whole process.

Parents and other family members can use dialogue journals to encourage writing and reading at home. The interactive element of the journals makes them a natural activity for use at home. They allow children to see that writing and reading are not just things you do at school. Children come to see that writing is a way of recording information, expressing feelings, and interacting with other people.

# Journal

*Ann,*

*Today I had a busy day, too, but I didn't get to make Rudolph the Red-Nosed Reindeer like you! I bet that really was fun! You are lucky!*

*Love, Mom*

*MOM*

*ON SattrDey I LOST MY tooth et SrPriD Me! He He Ha Ha I was SrPrisD wrreD AND HaPPY GOSH KLek It came owat I Bet IN Too A APPOLe AND et Kam AWt*

*Love, Ann*

(Translation of Ann's entry: "Mom, On Saturday I lost my tooth. It surprised me! He he ha ha. I was surprised, worried, and happy. Gosh, click. It came out. I bit into an apple and it came out. Love, Ann.")

*Ann,*

*You weren't the only one surprised when you lost your first tooth! I didn't think it was ready to come out yet, so it surprised me too! How does it feel to have an empty space in your mouth? Draw me a picture of what you look like now!*

*Love, Mom*

*Mommy It fels fane too Have a spas in my mawthe My ton ceps coming in lat plas I git tiyrd av les spas*

*Love, Ann*

(Translation of Ann's entry: "Mommy, It feels funny to have a space in my mouth. My tongue keeps coming in that place. I get tired of this space. Love, Ann.")

*Ann,*

*I love the picture you drew of yourself! I hope you soon get used to having a space in your mouth. Pretty soon you'll probably have more and more spaces! That will really look and feel funny! Tell me about your school day.*

*Love, Mom*

# Dialogue Journals at Home

Parents often ask teachers how they can help their child at home with schoolwork. What parents usually have in mind is how to help with homework. As an alternative, suggest using a dialogue journal. Explain to parents how keeping a journal provides regular practice in writing and, more important, it helps to build bonds of communication among family members. The child writes an entry, and then one or both parents respond. Brothers and sisters also can share dialogue journals. Even grandparents and other relatives who live far away can get in on the fun. A small spiral notebook with journal entries can be mailed back and forth at little cost. It is exciting for children to receive messages from relatives, who respond to the comments on events in a child's life.

Even very young children can participate in the interaction of a dialogue journal. Their journal entries may be drawings or simple messages written with invented spelling, but nevertheless they are communicating. Following are some excerpts from a dialogue journal kept by a mother and her kindergarten daughter, Ann, over a span of a few days. (For the reader who has difficulty comprehending Ann's invented spelling, a translation is provided.) In an earlier entry, Ann had written about the fun she had at school making Rudolph the Red-Nosed Reindeer. The first entry is from her mother.

Ron responds to the questions by writing short comments in the margin next to the teacher's journal entry. In a later entry, Ron questions the accuracy of the illustrations of Willy at the end of the book, after he has been through his body-building program, because they don't look any different than the illustrations of Willy at the beginning of the book. This kind of questioning shows the thinking Ron engages in as he reads a book.

Dialogue journals allow children to interact with one another and with their teachers on a broad range of ideas and personal insights about books they have read. This opportunity to share in writing makes reading more fun and, at the same time, gives children greater insight into what they have read.

*Tom,*

*I'm glad you liked the book. Could Willy have gotten strong without the book? What do you mean by: "Things like that don't always work"? Have you ever ordered something that wasn't really what you thought it would be? Thanks for sharing.*
— *Mrs. Danielson*

*1st Yes, alls he had to do is pushups and situps.*
*2nd Like on T.V. they avertize all that. And a lot of people say it don't work.*

Then Jeff writes about his reactions to Willy. The teacher's response prompts Jeff to think about things that make a person "wimpy."

### Journal

*I did not think Willy was a wimp but he acted like it.*

*Jeff,*

*Why didn't you think Willy was a wimp? Do you act like a wimp sometimes? I know I do — especially around snakes or mice. Does anything really scare you? Thanks for sharing.*

— *Mrs. Danielson*

*I like snakes and rats and mice. Why are you scard of snakes and mice? Because they are slimy and scratchy and sneaky (both)?*

Ron responds to the book in a different way by asking questions about the book:

### Journal

*Why did Willy say I'm sorry to the postman when he didn't get his pacage? How did the gang know that Willy was strong?*

*Ron,*

*I think Willy said he was sorry because he apologized to everyone, even when it wasn't his fault. Your second question is especially good! Willy looked like his old self in those pictures, didn't he? Maybe the gang heard that he had been working out and that's how they knew he was strong. Thanks for sharing.*
— *Mrs. Danielson*

*P.S. Did you like the book?*

their teacher can share their excitement about books and reading. At the same time, they are practicing their writing on something they really care about.

Following are journal excerpts about books read by students in a fifth-grade class. In the first excerpt, Tom writes his reaction to *Something Special For Me* by Vera Williams. In this book Rosa cannot decide what present she would like to receive for her birthday. She thinks about all sorts of ideas and finally decides on an accordion. Tom's journal entry and the teacher's response follow:

### Journal

*I thought it was like me in one way. I can never decide what to get. When I can't decide what to get I get mad and then I don't get anything. That's the way it is when I get shoes.*

*Tom,*
  *It is hard to decide on what to get. What happens to you when you get shoes? I was surprised that Rosa picked an accordion for her gift. Were you? Thanks for sharing.*

  — *Mrs. Danielson*

*I find a lot of shoes that I like and can't decide which pair to get!*

Another book, read by three boys, was *Willy the Wimp* by Anthony Browne — about a gorilla who apologizes for everything, even when things are not his fault. Willy is somewhat smaller than his peers, especially the suburban gorilla gang who continually threaten to beat him up. Following are journal entries by the three boys and my responses. Note the boys' varied reactions to the story. First, we hear from Tom again:

### Journal

*This story is good because he got beat up for a long time and then was tired of it, so he got this book that told him how to be big and strong and it worked. Things like that don't always work.*

# Dialogue Journals and the Reading Curriculum

One of the best ways of using dialogue journals is with books that children have read or with books the teacher reads to them. And they are a welcome alternative to the formal book report. Children usually have reactions to books that they read or that are read to them. The dialogue journal provides a relaxed way for them to write their reactions and opinions about books and to enjoy a response to what they have written.

Children can write whatever they want about a book. They can write their reactions about the characters and the plot while they read the book. For example, they might question why the author had a character do something that seems inconsistent, or they might conjecture as to what they think is going to happen next. If the teacher is reading the book aloud to the class over several days, she can set aside a few minutes after each session for the children to write in their journals. Students might write about what the book reminded them of or perhaps about a similar experience they have had. They also can write evaluative comments expressing their feelings about the book. If the book is a picture book, they can comment on the illustrations.

The collection of children's journal entries becomes a good source of information about what they like or don't like about certain books. By sharing journals with other children, they serve as good advertising for reading other books. With the journals, both the children and

The dialogue journal excerpts above do not cover topics of great importance. Rather, they are conversations in writing along the lines of "getting to know you." They build confidence in writing and they build friendships. They help to make our schools friendlier places.

Student: *I think that you are very perceptive. I do enjoy riding it, but sometimes, especially at 7:00 a.m., it gets to be more of a task than fun.*

Instructor: *Do your kids like to ride on it? I haven't been on a motorcycle for years. I think I'm scared to death of them, to be honest. Have you ever been on a three-wheeler? That's more my speed — although they can be dangerous too.*

Student: *My kids are always fighting over who is going to ride with me. No, I have not been on a three-wheeler, but I think that it would be fun. I like being outdoors, which is probably why I like riding my motorcycle.*

Instructor: *I'm sure your kids love it. A three-wheeler is kind of fun, but I'm not always sure what gear I'm in!*

Student: *List of three words — tired, dog, busy.*

Instructor: *I'm assuming you have a dog, or want one. What kind? I think my favorite dog is a collie. When we were kids, we had one named Manfred. Collies are so pleasant natured and independent. I like those qualities in a dog. What do you think?*

Student: *My roommate has two Scotties. They are really fun to play with. I take them for long walks. There's nothing like having a dog to talk with and walk with. The problem is they love people. Rather than being watchdogs, they are everyone's best friend.*

Instructor: *What are the dogs' names? Some dogs just don't make good watchdogs. What do you think about cats? I think cats are interesting to watch. I don't have any pets right now, because we live in an apartment that doesn't allow them. I must admit that I enjoy the quiet, though.*

Student: *The dogs' names are Dundee and Huntley. Dundee is a year old and Huntley is nine months. They're very fun and full of energy. I like cats, but I hate cat litter boxes. The cat hair is a real mess also. My boyfriend has two cats that are so fluffy and pretty.*

Instructor: *I like those names! I'll bet they fit their personalities. Cat hair is a problem. We used to have lots of cats on the farm when I was growing up. We were never too original with names, though — Blacky, Tabby, etc.*

Student: *I love animals. It is really interesting how names fit them. I had a bird once. I called her "Jaws" because she used to peck so hard when you would clean her cage. I had a kitten once, too. The kitten broke too many things, we had to get rid of him.*

The three-word journal also can be used to establish rapport between students or between a student and the teacher. The first two excerpts below are from journals of two sets of college students using the three-word technique. The last two are from a college student and her instructor.

## *Journal*

Student One: *Three words — pink, hungry, work.*

Student Two: *I am wondering if you listed the word "pink" because it's your favorite color. You are wearing pink pants and your blouse has a pink design. You look nice in pink, so you may enjoy wearing that color. Is there any other reason you chose pink?*

Student One: *Yes, pink is my favorite color. I used to have almost all pink in my wardrobe, but I got tired of it, so now I save pink for special days or days that I need an uplift. I hate pink cars, pink bathrooms and kitchens, and pink houses. Do you like pink?*

Student Two: *My grandma had a pink bathroom! I like pink, too, (clothes, that is) or a soft, warm, pink blanket.*

Student Three: *List of three words — black, middle, into.*

Student Four: *Lisa, why on earth did black pop into your mind? Are you depressed? Did you eat burnt toast this morning? Black is a very interesting color. Sometimes I like the color black because it appears to make me look thinner. How does black look on you?*

Student Three: *Black is my best color! I love it! Maybe it makes me look thinner too, I don't know. I want a black cat and a black dog. I also think black is neat because you can wear it when you're sad or happy.*

Student Four: *Lisa, on your wedding day did you wear black? Just kidding! I hope you get a black cat, black dog, and a black child! Ha! Ha! I tricked you didn't I?*

Student: *List of three words — tired, wheels, how.*

Instructor: *You ride a motorcycle, isn't that right? I'll bet you get tired riding from Seward every day. But maybe the trip to school/work and back home helps you to clear your mind. What do you think?*

The dialogue journal also can be the place for students to ask what they think are "dumb questions," which they are embarrassed to ask in class in front of their peers. Following are excerpts from the journals of two college students enrolled in an education course. Both had specific questions related to the course, which they felt awkward asking in class.

*Journal*

*How long does it usually take to receive a film, and how much does it cost? Do most schools have many films to pick from? These may be simple questions, but I have never ordered films and/or books.*

*Do you think that his fidgety behavior is normal for third-graders, or is it an area he needs help with in order to concentrate and listen better? And if so, what kinds of activities would be best to help with this? Or what is needed?*
*P.S. Sorry this is so long; my pen must have got stuck on go!*

A simple technique for getting students used to the idea of writing in a dialogue journal is called the "three-word journal." For example, after a class discussion on a given topic, the teacher might ask students to write down three words that they think summarize or are central to the discussion. The person responding (another student or the teacher) would then select one of the words and write something about it. It could be a question requiring a response, a comment, an elaboration of a point, or a personal observation. The purpose is simply to start a conversation in writing.

In a sixth-grade social studies class that is discussing the economy of the Midwest, a student might write the three words: Farming, Ranching, and Family. The teacher might respond in this fashion: "I'm interested that you included the word 'Family' along with 'Farming' and 'Ranching' in your list. Why did you include that word? Why is it important to you?" Or the teacher might elaborate on the word with these comments: "Family is important to me, too. I am married and have one brother and one sister. What about you? Do you have brothers and sisters?"

## Dialogue Journals in the Content Areas

Dialogue journals have many uses in the content areas. When reading a textbook or other reference work for social studies, students might write questions in their journals on concepts or terminology about which they are uncertain. Journals can be used similarly in the science class. Writing in their journals gives students practice in using the vocabulary and concepts of different disciplines, which reinforces content learning. (See fastback 209 *Writing to Learn Across the Curriculum.*)

Dialogue journals can be used in foreign language classes to promote fluency in informal kinds of communication. When students write in another language, they gain practice in the use of vocabulary and grammatical structures needed for conversation.

Dialogue journals have also been used successfully with deaf students. It provides them with a medium that compensates for the lack of oral communication imposed by their hearing impairment.

One of the best uses of dialogue journals is as a forum for students to comment on issues of the day. Students can write from their own experience and offer their own opinions about items in the news. Sometimes the teacher might want to direct students' journal writing by posing open-ended questions based on some event in the news that day. This can lead to some lively debate in writing if students with different points of view become journal partners.

person. This purpose is compromised if teachers insist on correcting students' writing. Resist the urge; save the corrections for other kinds of writing in which students expect to have their work corrected. This is not to say that a teacher should not model correct spelling, for example, when responding to a student journal entry. When students see a word they have misspelled on their entry spelled correctly in the teacher's response, they are likely to get it right the next time.

as well as with quilts. The reader can see the interactive nature of the journal as the conversation in print continues.

### Journal

*I would like to have a quilt like that. It would probably be warm since it's gone through so much. I thought it was a neat story. Our family has moved a lot, and we are finishing our house right now! My mom and dad say we are never going to move again.*

*Mary*

*Mary,*

*That quilt was beautiful! Where have you lived? Is your house that you are finishing in the country? Why are your parents tired of moving? (Actually, I think I know the answer to that!) I have lived in Nebraska all my life, but in different cities. I also lived in Yellowstone National Park for three summers. Moving is not fun.*

*Thanks, Mrs. Danielson*

*I've lived in Cheyenne, Wyoming, then my sister, my mom, and me moved to my aunt's house, while my brother, my other sister, and my dad stayed at Cheyenne. Then we all moved to a house near Hickman. Then we moved into a trailer, then we moved into our house. Our house is in the country.*

*My parents are tired of moving because they think it is too much of a hassle.*

Students can be journal partners with classmates or with friends in another grade. Teachers also can have journal partners with colleagues in the same or different grade levels. The journal provides a convenient format for voicing concerns; celebrating events; and sharing opinions about children, school policies, and outside interests.

The journal can be a standard looseleaf or spiral notebook, or students can make their own journals by decorating a cover and stapling sheets of paper inside. Journals also can be done on a computer word processor, with the students and the teacher writing their entries and responses on the disk to share at a convenient time.

The purpose of dialogue journals is to give students practice writing in a conversational tone and to share their writing with another

# Dialogue Journals in the Elementary Classroom

Dialogue journals can be used with children of all ages. Kindergartners can use drawings, scribbles, invented spellings, or a combination of pictures and words. If the teacher is unable to interpret the message, the children can "read" what they have "written." Dialogue journals used at this age level give children a sense of pride as they produce meaning through symbols. Teachers in turn have the opportunity to provide personal feedback to the children's messages.

When primary grade students use dialogue journals, their teachers can model correct spelling and usage and ask elaborative questions, which motivates the children to do additional writing. Also, teachers can write about their own life experiences as they respond to the children's messages.

Students in the upper grades are capable of writing longer entries in their journals, but sometimes they are not sure how to begin. To overcome this hesitancy, teachers can suggest possible topics and set aside enough time for students to write without pressure. At this level students' journal entries can be narrative, expository, or expressive. Any of these forms of writing lend themselves to responses by the teacher, which build rapport with the student writer.

Following is an excerpt from a dialogue journal between a fifth-grade student and the author. Mary is writing about the book *The Quilt Story* by Tony Johnston, which deals with moving to a new house

Also important is that students see their teachers' writing. By modeling the act of writing, teachers show students that writing is a lifelong activity that is useful and something that should be shared. Teachers learn more about their students by writing to and with them. Teachers also learn more about themselves through the act of writing in journals. Dialogue journal writing is reflective, allowing two persons to examine each other's opinions and ideas and at the same time providing an opportunity for feedback. Both the reader and the writer benefit from such interaction in print.

In this fastback, I shall describe how dialogue journals can be used at all levels and in various content areas. With the many samples of dialogue writing provided, the reader will be able to see how this form of natural writing can become an effective method of teaching the process of writing.

# Introduction

Writing at any level is a direct and forceful means of communicating to others, but it also can be a means for personal inquiry and for clarifying one's thoughts. Writing structures thinking. It is active and interactive, personal and public.

One form of personal writing that teachers are beginning to use is the dialogue journal. Dialogue journals are a functional form of writing, much like having a conversation with another person: the student writes an entry and then the teacher writes a response to the content of the student's entry. The teacher may respond by asking relevant questions, by making personal comments, or by answering any questions that the student has asked. With dialogue journals, a student and a teacher write to clarify points and to gain insight into one another's perceptions. Dialogue journals allow both the reader and the writer to take risks in print as they discuss issues relevant to both of them. They also allow for the development of a relationship between two people, who communicate in and through print.

Dialogue journals can be used in a number of different classroom settings and for a variety of purposes. But the essence of the process is the partnership that is formed as both parties participate in the development of the journal. The student and the teacher come to know each other on a more personal level; a special rapport is established as they engage in the process.